Intuitive Eating For Beginners:

Listen to Your Body's Hunger Signals and Attain a Healthy Weight

By

Brittany Samons

Table of Contents

Intuitive Eating For Beginners: Listen to Your Body's Hunger Signals and Attain a Healthy Weight

By Brittany Samons

Introduction

Weight loss is among the most difficult thing a person could undergo. It takes long, it requires a lot of patience, and it needs sacrifices, especially if you are hoping to lose some weight with the use of some diet fads.

Most of the diets available nowadays, however, are not only sacrificial but have slow effects, too. Often, being on a diet for so long renders the diet ineffective and that reverting from it could cause the person to regain the weight he lost.

Furthermore, most diets give a person the feeling of being deprived. This, when not addressed, results in psychological changes that could render future attempts to lose weight difficult.

Fortunately, there is a philosophy that could help reshape our view of weight loss: Intuitive Eating.

Included in this book are the underlying principles and the benefits of Intuitive Eating. This book will guide you in your journey towards intuitive eating and will

give you the benefits of this revolutionary philosophy
in nutrition.

Chapter 1. Health and Eating Habits

The conditions for human life on earth have been drastically changed over time. Human ancestors hunted for food because of a need to feed more than their craving for food. Over the years, the human body has evolved to have adapted both to this kind of activity and to this degree of food availability. The driving force of hunting is sustenance and survival.

This primeval human desire to sustain and ensure survival caused humans to have evolved the capabilities to arrive at effective solutions for ensuring survival. As the most intellectually complex creature, humans have devised elaborate systems and means to ensure survival and to sustain it. Among these developments are those that concern the production, storage and processing of food.

Over the years, things changed. Humans have evolved from creatures who feed to live to those that live to feed. The human civilization has already passed the barrier of survival and advanced the living conditions to such a degree that feeding becomes an indulgence more than a necessity.

A study conducted in 2012 reveals that more than half of Americans who participated in a survey reveal that they have trouble controlling or rectifying their poor eating habits. Furthermore, while Americans consume almost a third more of packaged than fresh fruits, it was revealed in a study that 1 in four Americans consume fast food every day.

Poor eating habits among Americans have been correlated with an increase in the average weight of Americans and have been linked to various deadly diseases such as cardiovascular illnesses and metabolic syndromes.

Bad Eating Habits of Most of Americans

As the number of people gaining weight steadily increases every day, so are the number of those seeking ways to shed pounds are. It is estimated that Americans spent as much as $147 billion in 2008 to shed excess weight. However, despite the multitude of equipments, medications, food compounds and even diet programs, people are still gaining weight.

The fats stored within the body (hence the weight gain and the accompanying illnesses) can only be acquired the excess calories that we take in. Before the technologies and sciences that helped improve the number of availability of food nowadays, excess calories or sugars in the bloodstream were never an issue. The amount of the caloric intake of our ancestors somewhat equals to the expenditure.

Nowadays, people and the mentality on food have changed. We have become indulgent, and we have improved food so much that it has even affected how we perceive and react to hunger. If we boil down the issue on food to its core, we will see that its causes can be traced back to our poor eating habits.

Homeostatis

Scientists agree that nature (or the universe) behaves in such a way that it favors state of lower energy. That is, all systems will continue to react or move either until its energy is dissipated, or it is made to halt (or rest) or until it enters a state of equilibrium and be trapped in an endless loop.

The same is true with the design of the human body. Operating inside the human body is a mechanism for life centered on a harmonious balance between all operations in the body with only one goal: to ensure survival.

Homeostasis is an intelligent balance. It tells the body when it is cold and instructs it to heat it up; it tells the body when it is in danger and activates thinking and movement-boosting mechanisms to assist fight or flee; and it tells the body when it is deprived of energy and encourages the desire to seek sustenance through food.

Over the years, however, we have become blind, deaf and numb to these various internal processes. Before, our body sends the prompt for finding food in the form of hunger. Now, we barely feel hungry because we have developed and nurtured the habit of eating even if the body does not need it.

Bad Eating Habits that Equates to Ruin

Poor diet is more than just a choice based on an internal craving. The reason why poor food choices is difficult to change is because we have given in to food cravings for so many times that the tendency has been reinforced into our minds and have been embedded into our systems becoming a habit that is difficult to break. The following food habits are among the causes of poor food choices. Although breaking out of the habit is possible, even though the journey may be filled with failures and difficulties, still, prevention is way better than cure.

Keeping Foods Around

This tendency is hardwired into our systems. In the old times when our ancestors were faced with difficulty acquiring food, they keep a stash for the future. Nowadays, however, various food preparations extend the shelf life of foods many times of their usual storage life before.

This is the problem, however. This fear and this almost autonomic desire to provide for the future have already been trivialized by the assured availability of food for the future.

This habit is particularly detrimental as storing foods, which you always see regularly with appearances, designs, and packaging optimized to activate the hunger response overburdens the logic and resistance part of the brain. Overtime, a person fighting to resist the temptations of food will be conquered and will give in. In a study involving workers who were allowed to gorge in on candies placed upon the table, it was found out that those who were exposed to the appearance of candies were 71% more likely to eat them than those presented with candies in opaque containers.

Skipping Breakfast

After eight hours of fasting during sleep is the most important meal during the day: breakfast. Although dieticians have advocated cutting on calories, this does not necessarily mean skipping on breakfast. Studies suggest that those who eat breakfast are those that are more successful in losing and keeping an ideal weight. Furthermore, those who do are more likely to supplement on nutrients as calcium, vitamins C and A, riboflavin, iron, fiber and zinc.

People do not generally feel hungry after waking up. Thus, breakfasts need not necessarily be the first thing a person does in the morning. However, one must not go for hours without filling his stomach with complex carbohydrates loaded in fiber and nutrients to keep himself going for the rest of the day.

Distractions during Eating

One of the worst of eating habits is to allow distractions to interfere with eating. Scientists have discovered that when you are not paying attention, you lose the ability to keep tract of the amount of the food you take in and end up over eating instead. A recent study established that playing a certain game in computer erases your (subconscious) memory of eating during lunch and end up consuming more during snacks later.

Eating Food Out of its Bag

Eating food without seeing the contents or the amounts of the food you have consumed tends to allow a person to overindulge. One way of ensuring that you have enough control over what you eat and how much of the portion you partake is to literally watch what you eat while you eat. This is also the reason why keeping a food journal is beneficial: it allows you to see the amount of food you consume and decide for your subsequent action.

Eating while Busy

While eating on the run may seem a wise move to conserve and maximize time, it is, however, a bad decision to make when you are losing or maintaining weight. Doing this is like eating with distractions only with the addition of stress hormones and adrenaline, which are more likely to cause you to splurge on food.

Chapter 2. Intuitive Eating Basics

Intuitive eating is more of an eating philosophy than just simply a prescribed eating behavior. It is an encouraged mindset and approach which could help strengthen one's relationship with his food, mind and body gaining full control of his entire hunger and eating mechanisms.

Intuitive eating teaches a person to respond correctly to the signals his body is giving him. This belief is founded upon the premise that the human body is designed and is built upon a harmony (state of equilibrium) that is capable of regaining the same state once the body undergoes trauma or stress (from food depravity or hunger, injury, etc.,). This state of equilibrium can be threatened by dieting and other forms of caloric restrictions. Thus, any form of dieting or the deliberate reduction for food) activates various physiological and psychological adaptive reactions that could potentially ruin any weight-loss attempts—or worse, a person could be made unhealthier in the future. Studies have revealed that during depravity (caloric restriction), series of biological and hormonal functions happen within the body which could undermine plans for attaining an ideal weight. Thus, messing up with the natural system of your body could end up to a physiological state the favors weight gain. A craving that has biological and hormonal causes is difficult to resist.

The primary rule of this discipline is simple: eat when you are famished and stop when you are stuffed.

Characteristic of Intuitive Eating

Unlike diets which are restrictive in some way, intuitive eating does not restrict a person from eating foods. Although there are diets, which allow a person to gorge in on any food that he wants, still, it requires to a person to restrict consumption of certain foods deemed bad for the health. The actuality is, these diets have some impacts either physiologically or psychologically, that could lead to weight-management problems in the future regardless of its initial performance.

Intuitive eating has three characteristics.

It encourages a person to eat as a response to a physiological need rather than as a means for emotional comfort. Intuitive eating suggests that a person eats whenever he is hungry or feels discomfort similar to or associated with hunger.

Rely on body cues for hunger and satiety. Intuitive eating encourages a person to be more sensitive to the cues of the body to signal that it needs to feed or to stop eating. It does not rely on any psychological manifestations such as comfort from distress and does not decide to splurge based on what he sees (i.e. if food is abundant or looks great).

Does not have any food restrictions. A person can eat virtually anything in an intuitive eating mindset. He is not given restrictions based on food categories or the bad effects of food. This mindset maintains that the body can provide the right cue for the preference for the right type of food. Furthermore, when we say that intuitive eaters do not have food restrictions, we mean that they are given unconditional permission to eat. That means that they are advised to shed the belief that some foods are good or bad, are allowed to eat what they really wand and are freed from the obligatory penance associated with an indulgence in foods considered to be bad for health.

Intuitive eaters do not benefit from the stress-free provisions on food and are more likely to include a diverse and varied class of foods in the diet. Moreover, because they imbibe a mindset that transcends food eating habits, intuitive eater benefit from improved self-esteem, which results in a more positive perspective and a healthier body, as well.

Chapter 3. Principles of Intuitive Eating

One needs to follow certain principles in order to benefit from this eating philosophy:

Accept that Diet is Not Necessary for Weight Loss

Any form of restrictive diet is not beneficial in the end and the initial observable weight loss is offsetted by the roster of its bad effects. Start to reject the mentality of diet and begin to shed this old belief gradually. You may be one of the many who has experienced one or many types of diet and failed. It is, also, highly likely that you are one of those who experienced a diet, lost weight for few months from it, but eventually reached your limit and decided to stop with the diet. Consequently, afterwards, you may have experienced gaining weight—sometimes more than the amount you lost—resulting in a much heavier you. You should arrive at a decision now that maybe the solution is not on those diets but on our minds and our mindset.

Respect your Hunger

Contrary to most popular diets and disciplines nowadays, this instructs a person to restrict on calories in order to lose weight, intuitive eating suggests giving in to hunger. Not only will ignoring hunger affect the way your organs in your body operate, it will also trigger a physiological response, which will increase your craving and cause you to overeat. Furthermore, the effect of restricting caloric intake on craving and hunger tend to last for days on end.

Intuitive eating does not encourage eaters to restrict their food consumption. Rather, they are advised to heed it. Hunger is our own body's way of informing of a need to feed. In a healthy individual with normal hunger response, hunger is only triggered at certain times during the day and during low energy states. In intuitive eating, a person is encouraged to act on his hunger by eating regularly during times when your body feels hunger. They are also advised to consume food up until the stomach is full (not stuffed).

Befriend your Food

You have hated some foods (some being extremely tempting and delectable) for no reason. With the right mindset, your attitude on food will be normalized in time. With the right attitude towards food, craving and hunger can be managed easily and naturally. Forgive your food. Give yourself permission to eat any food you want to satisfy your hunger. Depriving yourself of food or restricting your access to food only leads to uncontrollable hunger I the future. Indulge and allow yourself to eat even the foods you labeled bad for you. Overtime, without restriction, your body will not feel the need to overeat and indulge, and your natural relationship with food will be restored.

Chase the Mind Police Away

Deep within our minds is a refined version of us called the mind police, which prohibit certain sets of actions such as indulging in bad foods. Since you are adopting a new view on nutrition and food, which encourages that you do not curb your food cravings, these mind police are no longer necessary. Chase these mind police away. What you want is to allow the natural mechanisms of your body to take over and let the natural homeostatic design have its way. Controlling your body through series of rules will only cause it to retaliate and inflict vengeance with fouler effects.

Respect your Body's Signals

If you are hungry, eat. If you are full, stop—this is what you get if you reduce intuitive eating into its simplest form. Allow yourself to feed when you feel uncomfortably hungry. Whenever you feel the physical (not psychological) symptoms of hunger, give in. Do not control it or do something to avoid it. The more you avoid hunger, the more your body will encourage you to overindulge later. Moreover, when you are full, stop eating. It takes a while before the body can recognize that it is actually full so sometimes we tend to eat past our stomach's normal capacity. Thus, one is encouraged to eat slowly to allow this normal mechanism to take over.

Recognize your Satisfaction Factor

One of the most crucial factors that could greatly assist a person in controlling his cravings is the degree at which he enjoys the very experience of eating the food in addition to enjoying the food itself. This technique has been greatly used by Japanese to their weight-loss endeavors. The principle states that when you are eating something you truly desire and enjoy in an environment that is both appealing and relaxing, the amount of satisfaction that you acquire from the experience is greatly amplified giving you the capacity to feel full with less food. This is because stress and discomfort prompt the body to enter a crisis mode—in this mode, it will consume as much as it can and store energy in order to prepare against the worst.

Separate your Feelings with you're Longing for Food

Whenever you feel stressed, afraid, bored, lonely, anxious or angry, find ways to find comfort and relief from these emotions without resorting to food. Although consuming food releases chemicals, which can trigger the feeling of relief and satisfaction, this solution is just physiological and is hence temporary. The most effective way of getting freed from the grapples of these emotions which has dire ramifications on one's health and weight is to analyze your emotions and the cause of each. Furthermore, the chemicals released by the brain during eating will not protect you from these emotions for so long. Like any other drugs, your brain and your body get accustomed (desensitized) to its effects. Overtime, you will need frequent and prolonged eating to free you from emotional burdens. If you keep relying on food for comfort, the last thing that you will notice is that your body is entering into a state where weight loss is becoming increasingly more difficult as time goes by.

Respect your Body

You can only do so much to improve the appearance of your body and reform it to something that pleases you. In the end, your genetic makeup is still in command when it comes to controlling your weight, eating patterns, and the physiology of your fat burning and storage processes. When there is nothing you can do to further improve your appearance then stop there. Do not force yourself to adhere to strict diets that will only give you illness in the end. Being able to respect your body and shun your overly critical impression on yourself will remove the necessity to adapt systems that you cannot follow. It will also allow your body to heal and return to its natural state.

Indulge in Physical Activity

Remove your thought on your weight-loss goals and the calorie burning effects of exercise. Rather, focus on the act of exercise itself and allow yourself to enjoy it. The very act of exercise alone will give you a new feeling and benefit your goals towards weight loss. Focus on how the exercise makes you feel, too, such as its energizing effects in order for you to enjoy the activity more. Losing weight as a motivation for exercise is a risky one since weight loss does not happen at a fast rate that you could expect. Instead, focus on the other benefits of exercise. In an intuitive eating philosophy, weight loss is never the goal but rather one of the benefits one enjoys.

Nurture your Body and Spirit

Select foods that you like and which makes you feel better. You must remember that perfection in a diet is unnecessary to achieving a healthy body. Stick to a group of foods that you personally like (because of its taste) and include them in your diet. When you consume foods that you enjoy and nourish your body at the same time, you create a physiological condition

that is stable and balanced and can respond normally
to various physiological states.

Chapter 4. Intuitive Eating on Occasions

Peer and social pressures remain to be two of the most influential factors in our decision-making process. The ideas and expectations of others of us remain to influence our decision out of fear of various discomforts because of not adhering to the expectations of our group or society.

Our eating patterns, habits and beliefs are one of those. An intuitive eater could easily find difficulties when in social gatherings or parties if he does not know the right thing to do. Here are some of the tips one can perform to ensure that they do not over indulge during those occasions:

Remind yourself that you can have access on those foods anytime later whenever you want one. One of the characteristics of intuitive eating is that it allows eaters to eat what they really want. So if you are particularly attracted to a certain food but are doubtful of your ability to control because you are distracted, and then remind yourself that you can have the food later. Furthermore, remind yourself that your new mindset has removed you of some bounding conditions to eat food. If you want to eat roasted turkey, you can have one if you like whenever you like it even if it is not Thanksgiving Day. To give it more power, promise yourself that you will make yourself any food you want at any time of the year whenever you crave for it.

To be able to expand your freedom more (and to convince yourself further that you can have the food anytime you want), ask for the recipe of something prepared in a party that you love or would really like to enjoy in the future. If it is not a bother, you can even put off eating for later. Say you do not feel hungry yet, but you are particularly drawn to a dish, why not asks the hostess to reserve you something to take home later.

Do not allow yourself to become so famished. Because of the desire to eat enough, sometimes you put off eating just to save up for a special event or a party later. This is not a good idea; however, since hunger tweaks your impression of satiety and makes you over indulge later ripping you of the feeling of being in control.

Instead, act like what intuitive eating expects you to: eat whenever hungry and eat relative to your hunger levels. If you want to preserve your appetite for an event later, you can also eat just enough for you to still feel hungry after a while.

You can also eat something in order to momentarily relieve you of your hunger. You do not want to walk into the party with the desperate feeling of wanting to eat.

Be kind to yourself. There is a chance, still, that despite the first two steps, you still overindulge during a holiday or an event. In such case, forgive yourself. These occasions do not happen so often and that a day of overindulgence will not do any difference. Hating yourself will only cause you emotional discomfort, which could affect your whole intuitive-eating mindset.

Conclusion

You have just finished a book on one of the most revolutionary philosophies about eating and nutrition. Your concept of weight loss and nutrition may have been changed significantly by the information outlined throughout this book.

Although intuitive eating cannot be adopted overnight, your journey towards it certainly has started the moment you started reading this book. It is now time for you to enjoy the roster of benefits of Intuitive Eating included within this book by practicing it. Overtime, not only will you gain expertise on the subject, you will also be moved deeper into it affording you of various benefits that you will not enjoy in any diet or conventional weight-loss programs.

I want to personally thank you for reading my book. I hope you found information in this book useful and I would be very grateful if you could leave your honest review about this book. I certainly want to thank you in advance for doing this.

If you have the time, you can check my other books too.